GRAIN FREE RECIPES COOKBOOK NEW EDITION 2024

Over 60+ Easy and Tasty Delicious Free Sugar - Grain free Recipes, Healthy Diet Eating for Beginners

**BY
DR. OLIVIA FAMA**

Copyright© 2024 By DR. OLIVIA FAMA All rights reserved worldwide.

No part of this book may be reproduced or transmitted in any form or by any means, electronic or mechanical, including photocopying, recording or by any information storage and retrieval system, without written permission from the publisher, except for the inclusion of brief quotations in a review.

Warning-Disclaimer

The purpose of this book is to educate and entertain. The author or publisher does not guarantee that anyone following the techniques, suggestions, tips, ideas, or strategies will become successful. The author and publisher shall have neither liability or responsibility to anyone with respect to any loss or damage caused, or alleged to be caused, directly or indirectly by the information contained in this book

Table of Contents

Introduction: 6
    Why Grain-Free? Unveiling the Power of Ingredients 6
    Beyond the Cookbook: A Lifestyle Guide 8
    benefits of a grain-free diet 10
    Preface: Dr. Olivia Fama's Personal Journey into Grain-Free Living 13
    Seasonal Specials: A Symphony of Flavors Throughout the Year 15
    Ingredient Spotlights: Elevating Your Grain-Free Culinary Experience 18
    Cooking Tips and Hacks: Crafting Culinary Excellence with Ease 21
    simple and delicious 14-day meal plan for beginners venturing into grain-free cooking 26
    grain-free breakfast recipes 30
        1. Almond Flour Pancakes: 30
        2. Chia Seed Pudding: 31
        3. Veggie Omelette: 31
        4. Greek Yogurt Parfait: 32
        5. Avocado and Smoked Salmon Roll-ups: ... 33
        6. Spinach and Mushroom Frittata: 33
        7. Coconut Flour Smoothie Bowl: 34
    grain-free lunch and dinner recipes 36
        8. Grilled Chicken Caesar Salad: 36
        9. Zucchini Noodles with Pesto and Shrimp: . 36
        10. Cauliflower Fried Rice with Chicken: ... 37

11. Salmon and Avocado Nori Rolls: 38
12. Beef and Broccoli Stir-Fry: 39
13. Turkey Lettuce Wraps: 39
14. Eggplant Lasagna: 40
15. Shrimp and Avocado Salad: 41
16. Chicken and Vegetable Skewers: 41
17. Spaghetti Squash with Meatballs and Marinara Sauce: 42

grain-free snack recipes 44
18. Almond Butter Energy Bites: 44
19. Guacamole and Veggie Sticks: 44
20. Roasted Chickpeas: 45
21. Caprese Skewers: 46
22. Deviled Eggs with Avocado: 47
23. Smoked Salmon Cucumber Bites: 47
24. Crispy Kale Chips: 48

grain-free dessert recipes 50
25. Almond Flour Chocolate Chip Cookies: .. 50
26. Coconut Flour Blueberry Muffins: 51
27. Avocado Chocolate Mousse: 51
28. Raspberry Coconut Chia Pudding: 52
29. Paleo Banana Bread: 53
30. No-Bake Coconut Bliss Balls: 54
31. Berry and Mint Sorbet: 55

grain-free vegetable and salad recipes 57
32. Roasted Brussels Sprouts with Bacon: ... 57
33. Cucumber and Tomato Salad: 57
34. Zucchini Noodle Salad with Pesto: 58

35. Grilled Eggplant and Tomato Salad:....59
36. Avocado and Arugula Salad:...............60
37. Cauliflower Salad with Lemon Tahini Dressing:..61
38. Spinach and Strawberry Salad with Balsamic Vinaigrette:................................62
39. Asparagus and Tomato Salad:............62
40. Broccoli and Bacon Salad:..................63
41. Grilled Portobello Mushrooms with Balsamic Glaze:..64

grain-free soup and stew recipes....................65
42. Chicken and Vegetable Soup:.............65
43. Spicy Shrimp and Coconut Soup:........66
44. Beef and Vegetable Stew:...................66
45. Butternut Squash Soup:......................67
46. Turkey and Kale Soup:........................68
47. Cauliflower and Leek Soup:................69
48. Salmon Chowder:................................70
49. Tomato Basil Soup:.............................71
50. Lamb and Vegetable Stew:.................72
51. Mushroom and Spinach Soup:............72

grain-free smoothie and other drink recipes...74
52. Berry Almond Smoothie:......................74
53. Avocado and Spinach Green Smoothie:. 74
54. Tropical Coconut Chia Pudding Smoothie:..75
55. Cucumber Mint Limeade:....................76
56. Chocolate Coconut Protein Shake:......77
57. Golden Turmeric Latte:........................77

4***

58. Raspberry Lime Sparkler:...................... 78
grain-free sweet treat recipes...........................80
    59. Almond Flour Brownies:....................... 80
    61. Coconut Flour Lemon Bars:................. 81
    62. No-Bake Energy Bites:........................81
    63. Vanilla Almond Butter Fudge:..............82
    64. Pumpkin Spice Energy Balls:.............. 83
    65. Chocolate Avocado Mousse:.............. 84
    66. Coconut and Almond Bliss Balls:........ 85
Conclusion... **86**
    BONUS... 87

Introduction:

Embrace a Grain-Free Revolution in 2024
Welcome to the latest edition of our Grain-Free Recipes Cookbook, where culinary innovation meets wholesome living. As we step into a new year, the dawn of 2024, we invite you on a gastronomic journey that transcends the ordinary and redefines the way we approach our daily meals.

In this edition, we celebrate the art of grain-free cooking—a lifestyle choice that extends beyond dietary preferences to embrace a holistic approach to well-being. Whether you're a seasoned enthusiast of grain-free living or embarking on this exciting culinary adventure for the first time, our cookbook is designed to captivate your taste buds and inspire a fresh perspective on the nourishment your body craves.

Why Grain-Free? Unveiling the Power of Ingredients

As we curate this collection of delectable recipes, we delve into the incredible world of alternative flours, nutrient-dense vegetables, and ingenious substitutes that redefine the possibilities in your kitchen. Discover the artistry behind almond flour's delicate textures, the versatility of coconut flour, and the transformative potential of vegetables like zucchini and cauliflower.

Beyond the tantalizing flavors, embracing a grain-free lifestyle offers a myriad of benefits—increased energy, improved digestion, and a renewed sense of vitality. The recipes within these pages are not just delicious; they are a celebration of nourishing your body and elevating your culinary experience.

A Culinary Adventure Awaits: What's Inside?

This cookbook is more than a compilation of recipes; it's a culinary adventure waiting to unfold. From sunrise breakfasts to decadent desserts, each page is a testament to the diverse and satisfying world of grain-free cuisine. Whether you seek quick and easy meals for busy days or crave the joy of leisurely cooking on weekends, there's a recipe to suit every occasion.

Explore vibrant salads bursting with seasonal freshness, savor the comfort of hearty main courses, and indulge in guilt-free desserts that redefine the meaning of sweet satisfaction. Our recipes don't just cater to your palate; they invite you to become a creator in the kitchen, weaving a tapestry of flavors that resonate with your unique taste.

Beyond the Cookbook: A Lifestyle Guide

More than just a collection of recipes, this cookbook is your guide to a grain-free lifestyle. Throughout these pages, you'll find tips for navigating the world of alternative ingredients, meal planning strategies, and insights into the nutritional powerhouses that form the foundation of each dish.

Join us as we embark on a culinary revolution in 2024—a journey that transcends the boundaries of conventional cooking and embraces the vibrant, health-conscious world of grain-free living. Whether you're a novice or a seasoned chef, our Grain-Free Recipes Cookbook is an invitation to savor every moment, celebrate every flavor, and embrace a new era of culinary excellence.

Welcome to a year of vibrant health, indulgent flavors, and the joy of creating wholesome, grain-free masterpieces in your kitchen.

Let the adventure begin!

[DR. OLIVIA FAMA]
Author, Grain-Free Recipes Cookbook 2024

benefits of a grain-free diet.

A grain-free diet involves eliminating grains such as wheat, rice, oats, barley, and corn from one's regular eating habits. Advocates of grain-free diets often highlight several potential benefits associated with this dietary approach. It's important to note that individual responses to diet can vary, and consulting with a healthcare professional or nutritionist is advisable before making significant changes to your eating habits. Here are some potential benefits often associated with a grain-free diet:

Improved Digestive Health:
- Some individuals may experience digestive issues, such as bloating, gas, or irritable bowel syndrome (IBS), due to the presence of certain compounds in grains. Removing grains from the diet may alleviate these symptoms for some people.

Stabilized Blood Sugar Levels:
- Grains, especially refined grains, can cause spikes and crashes in blood sugar levels. A grain-free diet, particularly one rich in vegetables, lean proteins, and healthy fats, may contribute to better blood sugar control.

Weight Management:
- Some people find that a grain-free diet helps them manage their weight more effectively. This may be due to reduced intake of processed and refined carbohydrates, leading to lower calorie consumption and improved satiety.

Reduced Inflammation:
- Grains contain compounds such as lectins and gluten, which can trigger inflammation in some individuals. For those sensitive to these compounds, eliminating grains might contribute to a reduction in overall inflammation.

Balanced Energy Levels:
- The elimination of grains and a focus on nutrient-dense foods can contribute to more stable energy levels throughout the day. This is often attributed to a reduced reliance on quick-burning carbohydrates that can lead to energy crashes.

Improved Mental Clarity:
- Some proponents of grain-free diets suggest that eliminating grains can contribute to improved mental clarity and focus. This could be related to stable blood sugar levels and reduced inflammation, which may positively impact cognitive function.

Potential for Gluten Sensitivity:
- Individuals with gluten sensitivity or celiac disease must avoid gluten-containing grains such as wheat, barley, and rye. For these individuals, a grain-free diet is necessary to prevent adverse reactions and promote overall health.

Encourages Whole, Nutrient-Dense Foods:
- A grain-free diet often encourages the consumption of whole, nutrient-dense foods such as fruits, vegetables, lean proteins, nuts, and seeds. This can contribute to a more diverse and nutrient-rich diet.

It's crucial to approach any dietary changes with careful consideration and, if needed, seek guidance from a healthcare professional or registered dietitian. While some individuals may experience benefits from a grain-free diet, others may find that a balanced approach that includes whole grains works well for them. Individual responses to diet can vary, and it's essential to find an eating pattern that aligns with your unique health needs and goals.

Preface: Dr. Olivia Fama's Personal Journey into Grain-Free Living

In the quiet corners of my kitchen, where the aroma of spices and the sizzle of ingredients mingled with the warmth of shared moments, my culinary journey took an unexpected turn—one that led me to embark on the creation of this Grain-Free Recipes Cookbook. Allow me to share with you the personal journey and the inspiration that fueled the inception of this flavorful adventure.

A Healing Quest: The Genesis of Change

Years ago, I found myself at a crossroads, facing a health challenge that prompted me to reevaluate the very essence of nourishment. Conventional wisdom often leads us down well-trodden paths, but in my quest for healing, I discovered the profound impact that food can have on our well-being. The realization that grains, despite their ubiquity, were contributing to my health struggles became a catalyst for change.

In the pursuit of holistic wellness, I delved into the world of grain-free living—a realm where the vibrant hues of vegetables and the richness of alternative flours became my palette for both healing and indulgence. As I embraced this new culinary ethos, I felt a resurgence of vitality, a renewal that extended beyond the confines of my kitchen to touch every aspect of my life.

The Birth of a Cookbook: Crafting Culinary Alchemy

In sharing my newfound passion for grain-free living with friends and family, I witnessed the transformative power of these recipes. Each dish became not just a nourishing meal but a testament to the joy of savoring the flavors of real, unprocessed ingredients. The overwhelming positive response ignited a spark within me—a desire to bring this culinary alchemy to a broader audience.

Thus, this cookbook emerged as a labor of love, a compilation of recipes that have graced my own table and have the potential to enrich the lives of those who embark on this grain-free journey with me. It is my sincere hope that these recipes not only tantalize your taste buds but become the cornerstone of your own path to well-being.

A Celebration of Wholesome Living

Beyond the confines of restrictive diets, this cookbook is an invitation to celebrate the abundance that a grain-free lifestyle offers. It's a celebration of vibrant health, a tribute to the joy of creating in the kitchen, and an ode to the timeless tradition of gathering around a table to share nourishment and stories.

As you flip through these pages, envision yourself not just following recipes but partaking in a culinary adventure—a journey that transcends the ordinary and redefines the way we approach food. May this cookbook be a source of inspiration, a companion on your quest for wellness, and a reminder that, in every meal, we have the opportunity to choose nourishment that uplifts our bodies and spirits alike.

Welcome to a world where grains are not absent but transformed into something extraordinary. Welcome to the Grain-Free Recipes Cookbook, a testament to the magic that happens when we choose to nourish ourselves with intention and joy.

With gratitude,
Dr. Olivia Fama

Seasonal Specials: A Symphony of Flavors Throughout the Year

In the realm of culinary exploration, there exists a magical dance with the seasons—a waltz that harmonizes the freshest produce and the ever-changing palette of flavors nature provides. In the pages of this cookbook, we celebrate this dance with our Seasonal Specials, a collection designed to elevate your dining experience and connect you with the bountiful offerings each season unveils.

Incorporating Seasonal Produce: Nature's Palette in Your Kitchen

As the seasons unfold, so too do the vibrant hues and distinct flavors of fruits, vegetables, and herbs. Our Seasonal Specials are meticulously crafted to embrace this natural rhythm, inviting you to explore the exquisite array of seasonal produce. From the crisp, earthy notes of spring greens to the robust and hearty fare of winter squashes, each recipe is a canvas upon which the essence of the season is painted.

Imagine savoring the sweetness of ripe berries in a summer salad, or the comforting warmth of a butternut squash soup on a crisp autumn evening. The Seasonal Specials section of this cookbook is a journey through the farmer's market and the orchard, bringing the very best of each season to your table.

Offering Variations for Year-Round Indulgence: A Culinary Calendar

Life, like the seasons, is ever-changing. Our cookbook recognizes the dynamic nature of your culinary journey and provides variations for different times of the year. Whether it's the light and refreshing salads that accompany sunny days or the hearty stews that warm your soul during colder months, our Seasonal Specials offer a diverse array of options.

Each recipe comes with suggestions for adapting to the nuances of the season. Feel free to experiment with different herbs, swap in seasonal fruits, or adjust the cooking methods to suit the weather outside your window. This flexibility ensures that your dining experience is not only delicious but also attuned to the unique moments of the year.

A Symphony of Flavors, A Tapestry of Memories

In embracing Seasonal Specials, you embark on a culinary journey that transcends the ordinary. It's not just about what's on your plate; it's about capturing the essence of the world outside your kitchen and infusing it into every bite. As you explore these recipes, you'll find that the changing seasons become not just a backdrop but an integral part of your dining experience.

Welcome to a culinary adventure that echoes the rhythm of nature. The Seasonal Specials in this cookbook are an invitation to savor the flavors of the moment, to celebrate the beauty of each season, and to create a tapestry of memories that lingers on your palate long after the last bite.

May your kitchen be filled with the bounty of the seasons, and may each meal be a celebration of the ever-changing, ever-delightful journey through the culinary calendar.

Bon appétit!
Dr. Olivia Fama and the Culinary Team

Ingredient Spotlights: Elevating Your Grain-Free Culinary Experience

Embarking on a grain-free journey opens the door to a world of innovative and wholesome ingredients that redefine the art of cooking. In this section, we shine a spotlight on three key players—almond flour, coconut flour, and tapioca starch—unveiling their unique attributes, health benefits, and offering guidance on where to procure them and how to wield their culinary magic effectively.

1. Almond Flour: A Nutrient-Rich Powerhouse

Benefits:

- ***Nutrient Density:*** Almond flour is rich in healthy fats, protein, and essential vitamins and minerals, including vitamin E and magnesium.
- ***Low in Carbs:*** It's a low-carbohydrate alternative to traditional flours, making it suitable for those following a low-carb or grain-free lifestyle.
- ***Delicate Texture:*** Almond flour lends a light and delicate texture to baked goods, from airy cakes to crispy crusts.

Tips:

- ***Where to Find:*** Almond flour is readily available in most grocery stores, health food stores, and online. Look for blanched

almond flour for a finer texture in baked goods.
- **_Effective Use:_** Substitute almond flour for traditional flour in a 1:1 ratio in most recipes. It's an excellent choice for cookies, muffins, and pie crusts.

Coconut Flour: The Fiber-Rich Gem

Benefits:
- **_High in Fiber:_** Coconut flour is an excellent source of fiber, promoting digestive health and providing a feeling of fullness.
- **_Low Carb:_** It's lower in carbohydrates than many other flours, making it suitable for those managing their carbohydrate intake.
- **_Subtle Sweetness:_** Coconut flour imparts a subtle coconut flavor to dishes, adding a touch of sweetness without added sugars.

Tips:
- **_Where to Find:_** You can find coconut flour in the baking aisle of most grocery stores, health food stores, and online.
- **_Effective Use:_** Due to its high absorbency, coconut flour requires more liquid than other flours. Use it in combination with other flours or increase the liquid content in recipes for best results.

Tapioca Starch: The Culinary Magician

Benefits:
- **Gluten-Free Thickener:** Tapioca starch is an excellent gluten-free thickening agent, ideal for sauces, soups, and gravies.
- **Adds Chewiness:** In baking, tapioca starch can contribute to a chewy texture, making it a valuable addition to grain-free bread and pizza crust recipes.
- **Neutral Flavor:** Tapioca starch has a neutral taste, allowing the flavors of other ingredients to shine.

Tips:
- **Where to Find:** Tapioca starch is commonly found in the baking section of grocery stores, as well as in specialty or health food stores.
- **Effective Use:** Use tapioca starch sparingly, as it can be dense. It's often used in combination with other flours to achieve the desired texture in baked goods.

Culinary Alchemy: A Symphony of Flavors and Textures

Now armed with the knowledge of these grain-free powerhouses, let your culinary imagination soar. Experiment, create, and savor the delightful results as almond flour, coconut flour, and tapioca starch transform your recipes into masterpieces. Whether you're a seasoned chef or an aspiring home cook, these ingredients are your allies in crafting delicious, grain-free wonders that nourish both body and soul.

Happy cooking!
Dr. Olivia Fama and the Culinary Team

Cooking Tips and Hacks: Crafting Culinary Excellence with Ease

Embarking on a grain-free culinary journey requires not only creativity but also a repertoire of techniques to master the unique characteristics of alternative flours. Additionally, time is a precious commodity in the kitchen, and strategic hacks can turn complex recipes into manageable feats. Let's dive into essential tips for achieving the best texture with alternative flours and time-saving hacks to make your grain-free cooking experience both delightful and efficient.

Tips for Achieving the Best Texture with Alternative Flours:

Blend and Balance:
- Mix different alternative flours to create a balanced texture. For instance, combine almond flour with coconut flour for a blend that offers both moisture and structure in baked goods.

Add Binding Agents:
- Alternative flours lack gluten, a common binding agent. Enhance the texture by incorporating binding agents like eggs, flaxseed gel, or xanthan gum, especially in recipes that require structure.

Experiment with Ratios:
- Adjust the ratio of alternative flours to find the perfect balance. Some recipes may benefit from a higher proportion of almond flour for a moist and tender result, while others may require a combination of flours for optimal texture.

Don't Overmix:
- Overmixing can lead to dense baked goods. Mix the batter or dough just until ingredients are combined to avoid overworking the alternative flours.

Use Liquid Wisely:
- Alternative flours, especially coconut flour, are absorbent. Gradually add liquids to the recipe and allow them to absorb fully. This prevents the mixture from becoming too dry or too wet.

Hacks for Saving Time in the Kitchen:

Batch Cooking:
- Prepare large quantities of grain-free staples, like cauliflower rice or almond flour muffins, and freeze them in individual portions. This allows for quick, grab-and-go meals during busy days.

Prep Ahead:
- Chop vegetables, portion ingredients, and pre-measure spices in advance. Having a well-organized mise en place streamlines the cooking process and reduces prep time when you're ready to start cooking.

One-Pan Wonders:
- Opt for one-pan or one-pot meals to minimize clean-up and save time. Roasting vegetables alongside proteins not only imparts delicious flavors but also simplifies the cooking process.

Invest in Kitchen Gadgets:
- Time-saving tools like a food processor, high-quality blender, or an immersion blender can expedite tasks like chopping, blending, and pureeing, making your grain-free cooking experience more efficient.

Explore Pre-Cut Options:
- While fresh is fantastic, consider using pre-cut or frozen vegetables when time is of the essence. This can be especially helpful for ingredients that require extensive preparation.

Master the Art of Simplicity:
- Embrace recipes with minimal ingredients and straightforward techniques. Simplicity not only saves time but allows the natural flavors of the ingredients to shine.

Culinary Mastery Awaits: Balancing Precision and Efficiency

Armed with these tips for achieving the best texture with alternative flours and time-saving hacks, you're poised to become a grain-free culinary maestro. Experiment, adapt, and enjoy the process of crafting delicious, nourishing meals that fit seamlessly into your busy lifestyle.

May your kitchen be a haven of creativity and efficiency as you embark on this delightful grain-free culinary adventure!

Happy cooking!
Dr. Olivia Fama and the Culinary Team

simple and delicious 14-day meal plan for beginners venturing into grain-free cooking.

Day 1:
Breakfast: Scrambled eggs with spinach and cherry tomatoes.
Lunch: Grilled chicken salad with mixed greens, avocado, and a lemon vinaigrette.
Dinner: Baked salmon with roasted Brussels sprouts and cauliflower rice.

Day 2:
Breakfast: Greek yogurt with berries and a sprinkle of chopped nuts.
Lunch: Zucchini noodles with pesto and grilled shrimp.
Dinner: Beef stir-fry with broccoli, bell peppers, and snap peas.

Day 3:
Breakfast: Almond flour pancakes with fresh berries and a dollop of Greek yogurt.
Lunch: Turkey lettuce wraps with avocado, cucumber, and salsa.
Dinner: Baked chicken thighs with sweet potato wedges and steamed green beans.

Day 4:
Breakfast: Chia seed pudding with coconut milk and sliced strawberries.

Lunch: Egg salad lettuce wraps with cherry tomatoes.
Dinner: Spaghetti squash with meatballs and marinara sauce.

Day 5:
Breakfast: Smoothie with spinach, banana, almond milk, and protein powder.
Lunch: Tuna salad stuffed in bell peppers.
Dinner: Grilled steak with asparagus and mashed cauliflower.

Day 6:
Breakfast: Omelette with mushrooms, onions, and feta cheese.
Lunch: Shrimp and avocado salad with a lime vinaigrette.
Dinner: Pork chops with roasted acorn squash and sautéed kale.

Day 7:
Breakfast: Coconut flour waffles with mixed berries.
Lunch: Caprese salad with mozzarella, tomatoes, and fresh basil.
Dinner: Baked cod with lemon-garlic butter, served with sautéed spinach.

Day 8:
Breakfast: Cottage cheese with sliced peaches and a sprinkle of chopped almonds.

Lunch: Chicken Caesar salad with homemade dressing.

Dinner: Lamb chops with roasted root vegetables.

Day 9:
Breakfast: Frittata with mushrooms, spinach, and cherry tomatoes.
Lunch: Avocado and shrimp ceviche.
Dinner: Turkey meatballs with zucchini noodles and marinara sauce.

Day 10:
Breakfast: Almond butter and banana smoothie.
Lunch: Chicken and vegetable skewers with tzatziki sauce.
Dinner: Baked tilapia with a side of steamed broccoli and cauliflower mash.

Day 11:
Breakfast: Scrambled eggs with diced bell peppers and salsa.
Lunch: Spinach and feta stuffed chicken breasts.
Dinner: Beef and vegetable curry with cauliflower rice.

Day 12:
Breakfast: Yogurt parfait with sliced kiwi and crushed pistachios.
Lunch: Shredded chicken salad with mixed greens, strawberries, and balsamic vinaigrette.
Dinner: Grilled shrimp with lemon-garlic butter, served with roasted asparagus.

Day 13:
Breakfast: Smoothie bowl with mixed berries, coconut flakes, and chia seeds.
Lunch: Turkey and avocado lettuce cups with a side of carrot sticks.
Dinner: Baked chicken thighs with Brussels sprouts and sweet potato wedges.

Day 14:
Breakfast: Almond flour muffins with raspberries.
Lunch: Salmon and avocado nori rolls.
Dinner: Vegetable stir-fry with tofu and cauliflower rice.

Feel free to mix and match these recipes based on your preferences. As you become more comfortable with grain-free cooking, don't hesitate to get creative and experiment with flavors and ingredients. Happy cooking!

grain-free breakfast recipes

1. Almond Flour Pancakes:

Preparation Time: 15 minutes
Nutrition:
  Calories: 250 per serving
  Protein: 10g
  Carbohydrates: 8g
  Fat: 20g
Ingredients:
- 1 cup almond flour
- 2 eggs
- 1/4 cup almond milk
- 1 tablespoon coconut oil
- 1 teaspoon baking powder
- Pinch of salt
- Optional: Berries, maple syrup for topping

Instructions:
1. In a bowl, whisk together almond flour, eggs, almond milk, coconut oil, baking powder, and salt until smooth.
2. Heat a skillet over medium heat and lightly grease with coconut oil.
3. Pour 1/4 cup of batter onto the skillet for each pancake.
4. Cook until bubbles form on the surface, then flip and cook the other side.
5. Serve with your favorite toppings.

2. Chia Seed Pudding:

Preparation Time: 5 minutes (plus chilling time)
Nutrition:
  Calories: 180 per serving
  Protein: 5g
  Carbohydrates: 20g
  Fat: 10g
Ingredients:
- 3 tablespoons chia seeds
- 1 cup almond milk
- 1 teaspoon vanilla extract
- Fresh berries for topping

Instructions:
1. In a bowl, mix chia seeds, almond milk, and vanilla extract.
2. Stir well and refrigerate for at least 2 hours or overnight.
3. Before serving, give it a good stir and top with fresh berries.

3. Veggie Omelette:

Preparation Time: 10 minutes
Nutrition:
  Calories: 300 per serving
  Protein: 15g
  Carbohydrates: 5g
  Fat: 24g
Ingredients:
- 3 eggs
- 1/4 cup diced bell peppers
- 1/4 cup diced tomatoes

- 1/4 cup diced onions
- Salt and pepper to taste
- 1 tablespoon olive oil

Instructions:
1. In a bowl, beat the eggs and season with salt and pepper.
2. Heat olive oil in a skillet over medium heat.
3. Add bell peppers, tomatoes, and onions to the skillet and sauté until softened.
4. Pour beaten eggs over the vegetables and cook until set.
5. Fold the omelette in half and serve hot.

4. Greek Yogurt Parfait:

Preparation Time: 5 minutes
Nutrition:
 Calories: 220 per serving
 Protein: 15g
 Carbohydrates: 15g
 Fat: 10g

Ingredients:
- 1 cup Greek yogurt
- 1/2 cup mixed berries
- 2 tablespoons chopped nuts (almonds, walnuts, or pistachios)
- Drizzle of honey

Instructions:
1. In a glass or bowl, layer Greek yogurt, mixed berries, and chopped nuts.
2. Repeat the layers.

3. Drizzle honey on top and enjoy!

5. Avocado and Smoked Salmon Roll-ups:

Preparation Time: 10 minutes
Nutrition:
  Calories: 280 per serving
  Protein: 15g
  Carbohydrates: 10g
  Fat: 20g
Ingredients:
- 1 ripe avocado
- 4 slices smoked salmon
- Fresh dill for garnish
- Lemon wedges

Instructions:
1. Slice the avocado into thin strips.
2. Lay a slice of smoked salmon flat and place avocado strips on top.
3. Roll the salmon around the avocado.
4. Garnish with fresh dill and serve with lemon wedges.

6. Spinach and Mushroom Frittata:

Preparation Time: 20 minutes
Nutrition:
  Calories: 220 per serving
  Protein: 12g
  Carbohydrates: 5g
  Fat: 18g
Ingredients:
- 4 eggs

- 1 cup fresh spinach, chopped
- 1/2 cup mushrooms, sliced
- 1/4 cup feta cheese, crumbled
- Salt and pepper to taste
- 1 tablespoon olive oil

Instructions:
1. Preheat the oven to 350°F (175°C).
2. In a bowl, whisk eggs and season with salt and pepper.
3. Heat olive oil in an oven-safe skillet over medium heat.
4. Add spinach and mushrooms to the skillet and sauté until wilted.
5. Pour the whisked eggs over the vegetables and sprinkle feta on top.
6. Transfer the skillet to the oven and bake for 12-15 minutes or until the frittata is set.

7. Coconut Flour Smoothie Bowl:

Preparation Time: 10 minutes
Nutrition:
  Calories: 280 per serving
  Protein: 10g
  Carbohydrates: 25g
  Fat: 15g
Ingredients:
- 1/2 cup coconut milk
- 1/2 frozen banana
- 1/4 cup shredded coconut
- 1 tablespoon chia seeds
- Fresh fruit for topping

Instructions:
1. In a blender, combine coconut milk, frozen banana, shredded coconut, and chia seeds.
2. Blend until smooth.
3. Pour the smoothie into a bowl and top with fresh fruit.

Feel free to customize these recipes based on your preferences and dietary needs. Happy grain-free breakfasting!

grain-free lunch and dinner recipes

8. Grilled Chicken Caesar Salad:

Preparation Time: 20 minutes
Nutrition:
  Calories: 400 per serving
  Protein: 30g
  Carbohydrates: 10g
  Fat: 25g
Ingredients:
- Grilled chicken breast
- Romaine lettuce
- Cherry tomatoes
- Parmesan cheese, shaved
- Caesar dressing (grain-free)

Instructions:
1. Grill the chicken breast until fully cooked.
2. Chop romaine lettuce and halve cherry tomatoes.
3. Slice grilled chicken and toss with lettuce, tomatoes, and shaved Parmesan.
4. Drizzle with grain-free Caesar dressing and toss before serving.

9. Zucchini Noodles with Pesto and Shrimp:

Preparation Time: 15 minutes
Nutrition:
  Calories: 320 per serving
  Protein: 20g
  Carbohydrates: 10g

Fat: 22g
Ingredients:
- Zucchini noodles
- Shrimp, peeled and deveined
- Pesto sauce (grain-free)
- Cherry tomatoes, halved
- Pine nuts, toasted

Instructions:
1. Sauté shrimp until cooked.
2. Spiralize zucchini into noodles.
3. Toss zucchini noodles with pesto, cooked shrimp, cherry tomatoes, and toasted pine nuts.

10. Cauliflower Fried Rice with Chicken:

Preparation Time: 25 minutes
Nutrition:
   Calories: 300 per serving
   Protein: 18g
   Carbohydrates: 15g
   Fat: 18g
Ingredients:
- Cauliflower rice
- Cooked chicken, diced
- Mixed vegetables (peas, carrots, bell peppers)
- Eggs, beaten
- Coconut aminos (grain-free soy sauce alternative)

Instructions:
1. Sauté mixed vegetables until tender.

2. Push vegetables to the side and scramble eggs in the pan.
3. Add cauliflower rice and cooked chicken to the pan, stirring well.
4. Season with coconut aminos and cook until everything is heated through.

11. Salmon and Avocado Nori Rolls:

Preparation Time: 15 minutes
Nutrition:
  Calories: 320 per serving
  Protein: 20g
  Carbohydrates: 10g
  Fat: 22g
Ingredients:
- Nori sheets
- Smoked salmon
- Avocado, sliced
- Cucumber, julienned
- Pickled ginger & coconut aminos for dipping

Instructions:
1. Place a nori sheet on a bamboo rolling mat.
2. Arrange slices of smoked salmon, avocado, and julienned cucumber.
3. Roll tightly and slice into bite-sized pieces.
4. Serve with pickled ginger and coconut aminos for dipping.

12. Beef and Broccoli Stir-Fry:

Preparation Time: 20 minutes
Nutrition:
   Calories: 350 per serving
   Protein: 25g
   Carbohydrates: 12g
   Fat: 20g
Ingredients:
- Beef strips
- Broccoli florets
- Coconut aminos
- Garlic, minced
- Ginger, grated
- Sesame oil

Instructions:
1. Stir-fry beef in sesame oil until browned.
2. Add minced garlic and grated ginger.
3. Toss in broccoli and cook until tender.
4. Pour coconut aminos over the mixture, stirring well until heated through.

13. Turkey Lettuce Wraps:

Preparation Time: 15 minutes
Nutrition:
   Calories: 280 per serving
   Protein: 22g
   Carbohydrates: 15g
   Fat: 15g
Ingredients:
- Ground turkey
- Lettuce leaves (iceberg or butter lettuce)

- Bell peppers, diced
- Onion, chopped
- Avocado, sliced

Instructions:
1. Brown ground turkey in a skillet.
2. Add diced bell peppers and chopped onions, cooking until softened.
3. Spoon the turkey mixture onto lettuce leaves and top with sliced avocado.

14. Eggplant Lasagna:

Preparation Time: 40 minutes
Nutrition:
  Calories: 320 per serving
  Protein: 18g
  Carbohydrates: 15g
  Fat: 22g
Ingredients:
- Eggplant, thinly sliced
- Ground beef or turkey
- Tomato sauce (grain-free)
- Cashew cheese (grain-free alternative)
- Fresh basil, chopped

Instructions:
1. Grill or roast eggplant slices until tender.
2. Brown ground beef or turkey in a skillet.
3. Layer eggplant slices, meat, tomato sauce, and cashew cheese in a baking dish.
4. Repeat layers and bake until bubbly. Top with chopped basil.

15. Shrimp and Avocado Salad:

Preparation Time: 15 minutes
Nutrition:
  Calories: 300 per serving
  Protein: 20g
  Carbohydrates: 10g
  Fat: 20g
Ingredients:
- Shrimp, cooked and peeled
- Mixed greens
- Avocado, diced
- Cherry tomatoes, halved
- Cilantro, chopped
- Lime vinaigrette (grain-free)

Instructions:
1. Toss mixed greens with cooked shrimp, diced avocado, cherry tomatoes, and cilantro.
2. Drizzle with lime vinaigrette and toss until well combined.

16. Chicken and Vegetable Skewers:

Preparation Time: 30 minutes (including marinating time)
Nutrition:
  Calories: 280 per serving
  Protein: 22g
  Carbohydrates: 10g
  Fat: 15g
Ingredients:
- Chicken breast, cut into cubes

- Bell peppers, cut into chunks
- Zucchini, sliced
- Red onion, cut into wedges
- Olive oil
- Garlic powder, paprika, salt, and pepper

Instructions:
1. Marinate chicken cubes and vegetables in olive oil, garlic powder, paprika, salt, and pepper for at least 20 minutes.
2. Thread onto skewers and grill until chicken is cooked through and vegetables are tender.

17. Spaghetti Squash with Meatballs and Marinara Sauce:

Preparation Time: 45 minutes
Nutrition:
  Calories: 320 per serving
  Protein: 20g
  Carbohydrates: 15g
  Fat: 18g

Ingredients:
- Spaghetti squash, halved and roasted
- Homemade meatballs (ground meat, almond flour, herbs)
- Grain-free marinara sauce
- Fresh basil, chopped

Instructions:
1. Roast spaghetti squash until fork-tender.

2. Prepare homemade meatballs using ground meat, almond flour, and herbs. Bake until cooked through.
3. Scrape spaghetti squash into strands and top with meatballs, marinara sauce, and chopped fresh basil.

Feel free to adjust these recipes according to your taste preferences and dietary requirements. Enjoy your delicious and satisfying grain-free meals!

grain-free snack recipes

18. Almond Butter Energy Bites:

Preparation Time: 15 minutes
Nutrition:
  Calories: 120 per serving
  Protein: 4g
  Carbohydrates: 8g
  Fat: 9g
Ingredients:
- 1 cup almond butter
- 1/2 cup shredded coconut
- 1/4 cup chia seeds
- 1/4 cup honey or maple syrup
- 1 teaspoon vanilla extract
- Pinch of salt

Instructions:
1. In a bowl, mix almond butter, shredded coconut, chia seeds, honey or maple syrup, vanilla extract, and a pinch of salt.
2. Form the mixture into bite-sized balls.
3. Refrigerate for at least 30 minutes before serving.

19. Guacamole and Veggie Sticks:

Preparation Time: 10 minutes
Nutrition:
  Calories: 150 per serving
  Protein: 2g
  Carbohydrates: 8g

Fat: 13g
Ingredients:
- 2 ripe avocados
- 1 tomato, diced
- 1/4 cup red onion, finely chopped
- 1 clove garlic, minced
- Juice of 1 lime
- Salt and pepper to taste
- Assorted vegetable sticks (carrots, cucumber, bell peppers)

Instructions:
1. Mash avocados in a bowl and mix in diced tomatoes, chopped red onion, minced garlic, lime juice, salt, and pepper.
2. Serve with vegetable sticks for dipping.

20. Roasted Chickpeas:

Preparation Time: 40 minutes
Nutrition:
  Calories: 130 per serving
  Protein: 5g
  Carbohydrates: 18g
  Fat: 4g
Ingredients:
- 1 can (15 oz) chickpeas, drained & rinsed
- 1 tablespoon olive oil
- 1 teaspoon smoked paprika
- 1/2 teaspoon cumin
- 1/2 teaspoon garlic powder
- Salt to taste

Instructions:
1. Preheat the oven to 400°F (200°C).
2. In a bowl, toss chickpeas with olive oil, smoked paprika, cumin, garlic powder, and salt.
3. Spread the chickpeas on a baking sheet and bake for 30-35 minutes, or until crispy.

21. Caprese Skewers:

Preparation Time: 10 minutes
Nutrition:
  Calories: 100 per serving
  Protein: 4g
  Carbohydrates: 3g
  Fat: 8g
Ingredients:
- Cherry tomatoes
- Fresh mozzarella balls
- Fresh basil leaves
- Balsamic glaze for drizzling

Instructions:
1. Thread a cherry tomato, a fresh mozzarella ball, and a basil leaf onto small skewers.
2. Arrange on a plate and drizzle with balsamic glaze.

22. Deviled Eggs with Avocado:

Preparation Time: 15 minutes
Nutrition:
  Calories: 70 per serving

Protein: 3g
Carbohydrates: 1g
Fat: 6g
Ingredients:
- 6 hard-boiled eggs, halved
- 1 ripe avocado
- 1 tablespoon mayonnaise (grain-free)
- 1 teaspoon Dijon mustard
- Salt and pepper to taste
- Paprika for garnish

Instructions:
1. Remove egg yolks and place them in a bowl.
2. Mash egg yolks with ripe avocado, mayonnaise, Dijon mustard, salt, and pepper.
3. Spoon the mixture back into egg white halves.
4. Garnish with paprika.

23. Smoked Salmon Cucumber Bites:

Preparation Time: 10 minutes
Nutrition:
  Calories: 90 per serving
  Protein: 5g
  Carbohydrates: 2g
  Fat: 7g
Ingredients:
- English cucumber, sliced
- Smoked salmon
- Cream cheese (grain-free)

Instructions:
1. Spread a thin layer of cream cheese on cucumber slices.
2. Top with smoked salmon.
3. Serve chilled.

24. Crispy Kale Chips:

Preparation Time: 20 minutes
Nutrition:
  Calories: 50 per serving
  Protein: 2g
  Carbohydrates: 7g
  Fat: 2g
Ingredients:
- Fresh kale leaves, stems removed
- Olive oil
- Salt and pepper to taste

Instructions:
1. Preheat the oven to 350°F (175°C).
2. Toss kale leaves with olive oil, salt, and pepper.
3. Arrange on a baking sheet and bake for 12-15 minutes or until crispy.

Feel free to adjust these recipes to your taste preferences, and enjoy these delicious and satisfying grain-free snacks!

grain-free dessert recipes

25. Almond Flour Chocolate Chip Cookies:

Preparation Time: 15 minutes
Nutrition:
  Calories: 120 per serving
  Protein: 3g
  Carbohydrates: 10g
  Fat: 8g
Ingredients:
- 1 cup almond flour
- 1/4 cup coconut oil, melted
- 1/4 cup honey or maple syrup
- 1 egg
- 1/2 teaspoon vanilla extract
- 1/4 teaspoon baking soda
- Pinch of salt
- 1/2 cup grain-free chocolate chips

Instructions:
1. Preheat the oven to 350°F (175°C).
2. In a bowl, mix almond flour, melted coconut oil, honey or maple syrup, egg, vanilla extract, baking soda, and a pinch of salt.
3. Fold in grain-free chocolate chips.
4. Drop spoonfuls of dough onto a baking sheet and bake for 10-12 minutes.

26. Coconut Flour Blueberry Muffins:

Preparation Time: 25 minutes
Nutrition:
  Calories: 150 per serving
  Protein: 4g
  Carbohydrates: 12g
  Fat: 9g
Ingredients:
- 1/2 cup coconut flour
- 1/4 cup coconut oil, melted
- 1/4 cup honey or maple syrup
- 4 eggs
- 1/2 teaspoon baking soda
- 1/2 teaspoon vanilla extract
- Pinch of salt
- 1/2 cup fresh blueberries

Instructions:
1. Preheat the oven to 350°F (175°C).
2. In a bowl, mix coconut flour, melted coconut oil, honey or maple syrup, eggs, baking soda, vanilla extract, and a pinch of salt.
3. Gently fold in fresh blueberries.
4. Spoon the batter into muffin cups and bake for 18-20 minutes.

27. Avocado Chocolate Mousse:

Preparation Time: 10 minutes
Nutrition:
  Calories: 180 per serving
  Protein: 3g

Carbohydrates: 12g
Fat: 14g
Ingredients:
- 2 ripe avocados
- 1/4 cup cocoa powder
- 1/4 cup honey or maple syrup
- 1 teaspoon vanilla extract
- Pinch of salt
- Optional: Fresh berries for garnish

Instructions:
1. In a blender or food processor, combine ripe avocados, cocoa powder, honey or maple syrup, vanilla extract, and a pinch of salt.
2. Blend until smooth and creamy.
3. Chill in the refrigerator for at least 2 hours before serving.
4. Garnish with fresh berries if desired.

28. Raspberry Coconut Chia Pudding:

Preparation Time: 5 minutes (plus chilling time)
Nutrition:
   Calories: 120 per serving
   Protein: 3g
   Carbohydrates: 15g
   Fat: 6g
Ingredients:
- 1/4 cup chia seeds
- 1 cup coconut milk
- 1/2 cup fresh raspberries
- 1 tablespoon honey or maple syrup

- 1/2 teaspoon vanilla extract
- Shredded coconut for topping

Instructions:
1. In a bowl, mix chia seeds, coconut milk, fresh raspberries, honey or maple syrup, and vanilla extract.
2. Stir well and refrigerate for at least 2 hours or overnight.
3. Before serving, top with shredded coconut.

29. Paleo Banana Bread:

Preparation Time: 15 minutes
Nutrition:
   Calories: 160 per serving
   Protein: 4g
   Carbohydrates: 15g
   Fat: 10g

Ingredients:
- 3 ripe bananas, mashed
- 3 eggs
- 1/4 cup coconut oil, melted
- 1/4 cup honey or maple syrup
- 1 teaspoon vanilla extract
- 1 1/2 cups almond flour
- 1/2 cup coconut flour
- 1 teaspoon baking soda
- 1/2 teaspoon cinnamon
- Pinch of salt
- Optional: Chopped nuts for added crunch

Instructions:

1. Preheat the oven to 350°F (175°C).
2. In a bowl, mix mashed bananas, eggs, melted coconut oil, honey or maple syrup, and vanilla extract.
3. In a separate bowl, whisk together almond flour, coconut flour, baking soda, cinnamon, and a pinch of salt.
4. Combine wet and dry ingredients, then fold in chopped nuts if desired.
5. Pour the batter into a greased loaf pan and bake for 45-50 minutes.

30. No-Bake Coconut Bliss Balls:

Preparation Time: 15 minutes
Nutrition:
  Calories: 100 per serving
  Protein: 2g
  Carbohydrates: 8g
  Fat: 7g
Ingredients:
- 1 cup shredded coconut
- 1/4 cup coconut oil, melted
- 2 tablespoons honey or maple syrup
- 1/2 teaspoon vanilla extract
- Pinch of salt
- Additional shredded coconut for rolling

Instructions:
1. In a food processor, blend shredded coconut, melted coconut oil, honey or maple syrup, vanilla extract, and a pinch of salt until a dough forms.

2. Roll the dough into small balls.
3. Roll each ball in additional shredded coconut to coat.
4. Refrigerate for at least 1 hour before serving.

31. Berry and Mint Sorbet:

Preparation Time: 5 minutes (plus freezing time)
Nutrition:
  Calories: 80 per serving
  Protein: 1g
  Carbohydrates: 20g
  Fat: 0g
Ingredients:
- 2 cups mixed berries (strawberries, blueberries, raspberries)
- 2 tablespoons honey or maple syrup
- Fresh mint leaves for garnish

Instructions:
1. In a blender, combine mixed berries and honey or maple syrup.
2. Blend until smooth.
3. Pour the mixture into a shallow dish and freeze for at least 4 hours, stirring every hour.
4. Scoop into bowls and garnish with fresh mint leaves.

Feel free to customize these recipes based on your taste preferences, and enjoy these delightful grain-free desserts!

grain-free vegetable and salad recipes

32. Roasted Brussels Sprouts with Bacon:

Preparation Time: 25 minutes
Nutrition:
  Calories: 150 per serving
  Protein: 5g
  Carbohydrates: 10g
  Fat: 10g
Ingredients:
- Brussels sprouts, halved
- Bacon slices, chopped
- Olive oil
- Salt and pepper to taste

Instructions:
1. Preheat the oven to 400°F (200°C).
2. Toss Brussels sprouts and chopped bacon with olive oil, salt, and pepper.
3. Spread on a baking sheet and roast for 20-25 minutes, or until Brussels sprouts are golden and crispy.

33. Cucumber and Tomato Salad:

Preparation Time: 15 minutes
Nutrition:
  Calories: 80 per serving
  Protein: 2g
  Carbohydrates: 8g
  Fat: 5g
Ingredients:

- English cucumber, diced
- Cherry tomatoes, halved
- Red onion, thinly sliced
- Feta cheese, crumbled
- Fresh basil, chopped
- Olive oil
- Balsamic vinegar
- Salt and pepper to taste

Instructions:
1. In a bowl, combine cucumber, cherry tomatoes, red onion, feta cheese, and fresh basil.
2. Drizzle with olive oil and balsamic vinegar.
3. Season with salt and pepper, toss, and serve.

34. Zucchini Noodle Salad with Pesto:

Preparation Time: 20 minutes
Nutrition:
  Calories: 120 per serving
  Protein: 3g
  Carbohydrates: 8g
  Fat: 9g
Ingredients:
- Zucchini noodles
- Cherry tomatoes, halved
- Pine nuts, toasted
- Pesto sauce (grain-free)
- Parmesan cheese, shaved (optional)

Instructions:

1. In a bowl, combine zucchini noodles, cherry tomatoes, and toasted pine nuts.
2. Toss with pesto sauce.
3. Top with shaved Parmesan cheese if desired.

35. Grilled Eggplant and Tomato Salad:

Preparation Time: 30 minutes
Nutrition:
  Calories: 120 per serving
  Protein: 3g
  Carbohydrates: 10g
  Fat: 8g
Ingredients:
- Eggplant, sliced
- Cherry tomatoes, halved
- Red bell pepper, sliced
- Red onion, thinly sliced
- Fresh parsley, chopped
- Olive oil
- Balsamic vinegar
- Salt and pepper to taste

Instructions:
1. Brush eggplant slices with olive oil and grill until tender.
2. In a bowl, combine grilled eggplant, cherry tomatoes, red bell pepper, red onion, and fresh parsley.
3. Drizzle with olive oil and balsamic vinegar.

4. Season with salt and pepper, toss, and serve.

36. Avocado and Arugula Salad:

Preparation Time: 15 minutes
Nutrition:
  Calories: 180 per serving
  Protein: 3g
  Carbohydrates: 10g
  Fat: 15g
Ingredients:
- Arugula
- Avocado, sliced
- Cherry tomatoes, halved
- Red onion, thinly sliced
- Goat cheese, crumbled
- Walnuts, chopped
- Olive oil
- Lemon juice
- Salt and pepper to taste

Instructions:
1. In a bowl, combine arugula, avocado, cherry tomatoes, red onion, goat cheese, and chopped walnuts.
2. Drizzle with olive oil and lemon juice.
3. Season with salt and pepper, toss, and serve.

37. Cauliflower Salad with Lemon Tahini Dressing:

Preparation Time: 20 minutes
Nutrition:
　Calories: 120 per serving
　Protein: 4g
　Carbohydrates: 8g
　Fat: 8g
Ingredients:
- Cauliflower florets, steamed
- Chickpeas, drained and rinsed
- Cucumber, diced
- Red bell pepper, diced
- Red onion, finely chopped
- Fresh parsley, chopped
- Tahini dressing (grain-free)
- Lemon zest
- Salt and pepper to taste

Instructions:
1. In a bowl, combine cauliflower florets, chickpeas, cucumber, red bell pepper, red onion, and fresh parsley.
2. Drizzle with tahini dressing.
3. Sprinkle lemon zest, season with salt and pepper, toss, and serve.

38. Spinach and Strawberry Salad with Balsamic Vinaigrette:

Preparation Time: 15 minutes
Nutrition:
 Calories: 100 per serving
 Protein: 3g
 Carbohydrates: 10g
 Fat: 6g
Ingredients:
- Fresh spinach leaves
- Strawberries, sliced
- Feta cheese, crumbled
- Red onion, thinly sliced
- Candied pecans, chopped
- Balsamic vinaigrette (grain-free)

Instructions:
1. In a bowl, combine fresh spinach, sliced strawberries, crumbled feta cheese, red onion, and candied pecans.
2. Drizzle with balsamic vinaigrette, toss, and serve.

39. Asparagus and Tomato Salad:

Preparation Time: 20 minutes
Nutrition:
 Calories: 80 per serving
 Protein: 3g
 Carbohydrates: 10g
 Fat: 4g
Ingredients:

- Asparagus spears, blanched
- Cherry tomatoes, halved
- Kalamata olives, sliced
- Red onion, thinly sliced
- Feta cheese, crumbled
- Olive oil
- Lemon juice
- Fresh oregano, chopped
- Salt and pepper to taste

Instructions:
1. In a bowl, combine blanched asparagus, cherry tomatoes, Kalamata olives, red onion, and crumbled feta cheese.
2. Drizzle with olive oil and lemon juice.
3. Sprinkle fresh oregano, season with salt and pepper, toss, and serve.

40. Broccoli and Bacon Salad:

Preparation Time: 20 minutes
Nutrition:
  Calories: 120 per serving
  Protein: 5g
  Carbohydrates: 8g
  Fat: 8g
Ingredients:
- Broccoli florets, blanched
- Bacon slices, cooked and crumbled
- Red grapes, halved
- Red onion, finely chopped
- Sunflower seeds
- Greek yogurt dressing (grain-free)

Instructions:
1. In a bowl, combine blanched broccoli florets, crumbled bacon, red grapes, red onion, and sunflower seeds.
2. Toss with Greek yogurt dressing and serve.

41. Grilled Portobello Mushrooms with Balsamic Glaze:

Preparation Time: 15 minutes
Nutrition:
  Calories: 90 per serving
  Protein: 4g
  Carbohydrates: 8g
  Fat: 6g
Ingredients:
- Portobello mushrooms, stems removed
- Olive oil
- Balsamic glaze
- Fresh thyme leaves
- Salt and pepper to taste

Instructions:
1. Brush Portobello mushrooms with olive oil and season with salt and pepper.
2. Grill until tender.
3. Drizzle with balsamic glaze and sprinkle fresh thyme leaves before serving.

Feel free to customize these recipes based on your taste preferences, and enjoy these nutritious and delicious grain-free vegetable and salad options!

grain-free soup and stew recipes

42. Chicken and Vegetable Soup:

Preparation Time: 30 minutes
Nutrition:
  Calories: 180 per serving
  Protein: 15g
  Carbohydrates: 10g
  Fat: 8g
Ingredients:
- Chicken breast, cooked and shredded
- Carrots, sliced
- Celery, chopped
- Onion, diced
- Garlic, minced
- Chicken broth (grain-free)
- Fresh thyme
- Salt and pepper to taste

Instructions:
1. Sauté onions and garlic until softened.
2. Add carrots, celery, and shredded chicken.
3. Pour in chicken broth, add fresh thyme, and season with salt and pepper.
4. Simmer until vegetables are tender.

43. Spicy Shrimp and Coconut Soup:

Preparation Time: 25 minutes
Nutrition:
  Calories: 220 per serving

Protein: 18g
Carbohydrates: 8g
Fat: 14g
Ingredients:
- Shrimp, peeled and deveined
- Coconut milk
- Red curry paste
- Fish sauce
- Lime juice
- Zucchini, spiralized
- Cilantro, chopped
- Red chili flakes (optional)

Instructions:
1. In a pot, combine coconut milk, red curry paste, fish sauce, and lime juice.
2. Add shrimp and zucchini noodles.
3. Simmer until shrimp are cooked.
4. Garnish with chopped cilantro and red chili flakes if desired.

44. Beef and Vegetable Stew:

Preparation Time: 40 minutes
Nutrition:
   Calories: 250 per serving
   Protein: 20g
   Carbohydrates: 12g
   Fat: 12g
Ingredients:
- Stew beef, cubed
- Sweet potatoes, diced
- Carrots, sliced

- Onion, diced
- Beef broth (grain-free)
- Tomato paste
- Garlic, minced
- Thyme and rosemary
- Salt and pepper to taste

Instructions:
1. Brown beef cubes in a pot.
2. Add diced sweet potatoes, sliced carrots, diced onion, and minced garlic.
3. Pour in beef broth, add tomato paste, thyme, rosemary, salt, and pepper.
4. Simmer until meat and vegetables are tender.

45. Butternut Squash Soup:

Preparation Time: 35 minutes
Nutrition:
   Calories: 180 per serving
   Protein: 4g
   Carbohydrates: 20g
   Fat: 10g
Ingredients:
- Butternut squash, peeled and cubed
- Onion, chopped
- Coconut oil
- Chicken or vegetable broth (grain-free)
- Ground cinnamon and nutmeg
- Salt and pepper to taste
- Coconut cream for garnish

Instructions:
1. Sauté chopped onions in coconut oil until translucent.
2. Add cubed butternut squash and broth.
3. Simmer until squash is tender, then blend until smooth.
4. Season with cinnamon, nutmeg, salt, and pepper.
5. Garnish with a swirl of coconut cream.

46. Turkey and Kale Soup:

Preparation Time: 30 minutes
Nutrition:
   Calories: 200 per serving
   Protein: 18g
   Carbohydrates: 10g
   Fat: 9g
Ingredients:
- Ground turkey
- Kale, chopped
- Carrots, sliced
- Garlic, minced
- Chicken broth (grain-free)
- Italian seasoning
- Salt and pepper to taste

Instructions:
1. Brown ground turkey in a pot.
2. Add chopped kale, sliced carrots, minced garlic, and chicken broth.
3. Season with Italian seasoning, salt, and pepper.

4. Simmer until vegetables are tender.

47. Cauliflower and Leek Soup:

Preparation Time: 25 minutes
Nutrition:
  Calories: 150 per serving
  Protein: 5g
  Carbohydrates: 10g
  Fat: 10g
Ingredients:
- Cauliflower, chopped
- Leeks, sliced
- Chicken or vegetable broth (grain-free)
- Coconut milk
- Garlic, minced
- Olive oil
- Fresh thyme
- Salt and pepper to taste

Instructions:
1. Sauté leeks and minced garlic in olive oil until softened.
2. Add chopped cauliflower, chicken or vegetable broth, and coconut milk.
3. Simmer until cauliflower is tender, then blend until smooth.
4. Season with fresh thyme, salt, and pepper.

48. Salmon Chowder:

Preparation Time: 30 minutes
Nutrition:
  Calories: 220 per serving
  Protein: 18g
  Carbohydrates: 12g
  Fat: 12g
Ingredients:
- Salmon fillets, diced
- Cauliflower florets, chopped
- Celery, chopped
- Onion, diced
- Chicken or vegetable broth (grain-free)
- Coconut milk
- Dill, chopped
- Salt and pepper to taste

Instructions:
1. Sauté diced onions and chopped celery until softened.
2. Add diced salmon, chopped cauliflower, chicken or vegetable broth, and coconut milk.
3. Simmer until salmon is cooked and cauliflower is tender.
4. Season with chopped dill, salt, and pepper.

49. Tomato Basil Soup:

Preparation Time: 25 minutes
Nutrition:
  Calories: 160 per serving

Protein: 5g
Carbohydrates: 12g
Fat: 10g
Ingredients:
- Tomatoes, chopped
- Onion, diced
- Garlic, minced
- Chicken or vegetable broth (grain-free)
- Fresh basil, chopped
- Olive oil
- Salt and pepper to taste
- Coconut cream for garnish

Instructions:
1. Sauté diced onions and minced garlic in olive oil until softened.
2. Add chopped tomatoes and chicken or vegetable broth.
3. Simmer until tomatoes are soft, then blend until smooth.
4. Stir in chopped basil, salt, and pepper.
5. Garnish with a dollop of coconut cream.

50. Lamb and Vegetable Stew:

Preparation Time: 40 minutes
Nutrition:
  Calories: 280 per serving
  Protein: 20g
  Carbohydrates: 15g
  Fat: 15g
Ingredients:
- Lamb stew meat, cubed

- Carrots, sliced
- Turnips, diced
- Onion, diced
- Beef broth (grain-free)
- Tomato paste
- Rosemary and thyme
- Salt and pepper to taste

Instructions:
1. Brown lamb cubes in a pot.
2. Add sliced carrots, diced turnips, diced onion, beef broth, and tomato paste.
3. Season with rosemary, thyme, salt, and pepper.
4. Simmer until meat and vegetables are tender.

51. Mushroom and Spinach Soup:

Preparation Time: 25 minutes
Nutrition:
 Calories: 140 per serving
 Protein: 6g
 Carbohydrates: 8g
 Fat: 10g
Ingredients:
- Mushrooms, sliced
- Fresh spinach leaves
- Onion, diced
- Garlic, minced
- Chicken or vegetable broth (grain-free)
- Coconut milk
- Thyme, chopped

- Salt and pepper to taste

Instructions:
1. Sauté diced onions and minced garlic until softened.
2. Add sliced mushrooms and cook until they release their moisture.
3. Pour in chicken or vegetable broth and coconut milk.
4. Add fresh spinach and chopped thyme.
5. Simmer until mushrooms are tender.

Feel free to adjust these recipes according to your taste preferences and dietary needs. Enjoy these delicious and hearty grain-free soups and stews!

grain-free smoothie and other drink recipes

52. Berry Almond Smoothie:

Preparation Time: 5 minutes
Nutrition:
   Calories: 180 per serving
   Protein: 6g
   Carbohydrates: 20g
   Fat: 9g
Ingredients:
- 1 cup mixed berries (strawberries, blueberries, raspberries)
- 1/2 banana
- 1 cup almond milk (unsweetened)
- 2 tablespoons almond butter
- Ice cubes

Instructions:
1. In a blender, combine mixed berries, banana, almond milk, and almond butter.
2. Blend until smooth.
3. Add ice cubes and blend again until desired consistency.

53. Avocado and Spinach Green Smoothie:

Preparation Time: 7 minutes
Nutrition:
   Calories: 200 per serving
   Protein: 7g
   Carbohydrates: 15g

Fat: 12g
Ingredients:
- 1/2 avocado
- Handful of spinach leaves
- 1/2 cup cucumber, sliced
- 1/2 green apple, cored and chopped
- 1 cup coconut water (unsweetened)
- Juice of 1 lime
- Ice cubes

Instructions:
1. In a blender, combine avocado, spinach, cucumber, green apple, coconut water, and lime juice.
2. Blend until smooth.
3. Add ice cubes and blend again until desired consistency.

54. Tropical Coconut Chia Pudding Smoothie:

Preparation Time: 10 minutes (plus chilling time for chia pudding)
Nutrition:
  Calories: 220 per serving
  Protein: 8g
  Carbohydrates: 25g
  Fat: 10g
Ingredients:
- 2 tablespoons chia seeds
- 1/2 cup coconut milk (unsweetened)
- 1/2 cup pineapple chunks
- 1/2 mango, peeled and diced

- 1/2 banana
- 1 cup coconut water (unsweetened)
- Ice cubes

Instructions:
1. Mix chia seeds with coconut milk and let it chill in the refrigerator for at least 2 hours or overnight.
2. In a blender, combine chia pudding, pineapple chunks, mango, banana, coconut water, and ice cubes.
3. Blend until smooth.

55. Cucumber Mint Limeade:

Preparation Time: 10 minutes
Nutrition:
  Calories: 40 per serving
  Protein: 1g
  Carbohydrates: 10g
  Fat: 0g
Ingredients:
- 1 cucumber, sliced
- Handful of fresh mint leaves
- Juice of 3 limes
- 1-2 tablespoons honey or maple syrup (optional)
- 4 cups water
- Ice cubes

Instructions:
1. In a pitcher, combine cucumber slices, fresh mint leaves, lime juice, and honey or maple syrup if desired.

2. Add water and stir well.
3. Refrigerate for at least 1 hour.
4. Serve over ice.

56. Chocolate Coconut Protein Shake:

Preparation Time: 5 minutes
Nutrition:
  Calories: 220 per serving
  Protein: 20g
  Carbohydrates: 10g
  Fat: 12g
Ingredients:
- 1 cup coconut milk (unsweetened)
- 1 scoop chocolate protein powder (grain-free)
- 1 tablespoon almond butter
- 1/2 teaspoon vanilla extract
- Ice cubes

Instructions:
1. In a blender, combine coconut milk, chocolate protein powder, almond butter, and vanilla extract.
2. Blend until smooth.
3. Add ice cubes and blend again until desired consistency.

57. Golden Turmeric Latte:

Preparation Time: 8 minutes
Nutrition:
  Calories: 120 per serving
  Protein: 2g

Carbohydrates: 10g
Fat: 8g
Ingredients:
- 1 cup almond milk (unsweetened)
- 1 teaspoon ground turmeric
- 1/2 teaspoon ground cinnamon
- 1/4 teaspoon ground ginger
- Pinch of black pepper
- 1 teaspoon honey or maple syrup (optional)
- Coconut oil for added creaminess

Instructions
1. In a small saucepan, heat almond milk, turmeric, cinnamon, ginger, black pepper, and honey or maple syrup over medium heat.
2. Whisk until well combined and heated through.
3. Pour into a mug, add a small amount of coconut oil for added creaminess, and stir.

58. Raspberry Lime Sparkler:

Preparation Time: 5 minutes
Nutrition:
  Calories: 60 per serving
  Protein: 1g
  Carbohydrates: 15g
  Fat: 0g
Ingredients:
- 1/2 cup fresh raspberries
- Juice of 2 limes

- 1 tablespoon honey or maple syrup
- Sparkling water
- Ice cubes
- Fresh mint for garnish

Instructions:
1. In a glass, muddle fresh raspberries with lime juice and honey or maple syrup.
2. Fill the glass with ice cubes.
3. Top with sparkling water and stir gently.
4. Garnish with fresh mint.

Feel free to customize these recipes based on your taste preferences and dietary needs. Enjoy these refreshing and nutritious grain-free smoothies and drinks!

grain-free sweet treat recipes

59. Almond Flour Brownies:

Preparation Time: 20 minutes
Nutrition:
  Calories: 150 per serving
  Protein: 4g
  Carbohydrates: 12g
  Fat: 10g
Ingredients:
- 1 cup almond flour
- 1/2 cup cocoa powder
- 1/2 cup coconut oil, melted
- 1 cup coconut sugar
- 2 large eggs
- 1 teaspoon vanilla extract
- 1/4 teaspoon baking soda
- Pinch of salt
- 1/2 cup chopped nuts or grain-free chocolate chips (optional)

Instructions:
1. Preheat the oven to 350°F (175°C).
2. In a bowl, mix almond flour, cocoa powder, melted coconut oil, coconut sugar, eggs, vanilla extract, baking soda, and salt.
3. Fold in chopped nuts or chocolate chips if desired.
4. Spread the batter into a greased baking dish and bake for 20-25 minutes.

61. Coconut Flour Lemon Bars:

Preparation Time: 25 minutes
Nutrition:
  Calories: 120 per serving
  Protein: 3g
  Carbohydrates: 10g
  Fat: 8g
Ingredients:
- 1/2 cup coconut flour
- 1/2 cup coconut oil, melted
- 1/4 cup honey or maple syrup
- 4 eggs
- Zest and juice of 2 lemons
- 1/2 teaspoon baking soda
- Pinch of salt

Instructions:
1. Preheat the oven to 350°F (175°C).
2. In a bowl, mix coconut flour, melted coconut oil, honey or maple syrup, eggs, lemon zest, lemon juice, baking soda, and salt.
3. Pour the batter into a greased baking dish and bake for 18-20 minutes.
4. Allow to cool before cutting into bars.

62. No-Bake Energy Bites:

Preparation Time: 15 minutes
Nutrition:
  Calories: 100 per serving
  Protein: 4g
  Carbohydrates: 8g

Fat: 6g
Ingredients:
- 1 cup almond flour
- 1/2 cup nut butter (almond, peanut, or cashew)
- 1/4 cup honey or maple syrup
- 1/2 cup shredded coconut
- 1/2 cup chopped nuts or seeds (e.g., almonds, sunflower seeds)
- 1 teaspoon vanilla extract
- Pinch of salt
- Additional shredded coconut for rolling

Instructions:
1. In a bowl, combine almond flour, nut butter, honey or maple syrup, shredded coconut, chopped nuts or seeds, vanilla extract, and salt.
2. Mix until well combined.
3. Roll the mixture into small balls and coat with additional shredded coconut.
4. Refrigerate for at least 1 hour before serving.

63. Vanilla Almond Butter Fudge:

Preparation Time: 15 minutes
Nutrition:
　Calories: 160 per serving
　Protein: 4g
　Carbohydrates: 10g
　Fat: 12g
Ingredients:

- 1 cup almond butter
- 1/4 cup coconut oil, melted
- 1/4 cup honey or maple syrup
- 1 teaspoon vanilla extract
- Pinch of salt

Instructions:
1. In a bowl, mix almond butter, melted coconut oil, honey or maple syrup, vanilla extract, and salt.
2. Pour the mixture into a lined baking dish.
3. Freeze for at least 2 hours, then cut into squares before serving.

64. Pumpkin Spice Energy Balls:

Preparation Time: 15 minutes
Nutrition:
   Calories: 120 per serving
   Protein: 3g
   Carbohydrates: 10g
   Fat: 8g
Ingredients:
- 1 cup almond flour
- 1/4 cup pumpkin puree
- 1/4 cup almond butter
- 2 tablespoons honey or maple syrup
- 1 teaspoon pumpkin spice blend
- Pinch of salt
- Chopped pecans for coating (optional)

Instructions:

1. In a bowl, combine almond flour, pumpkin puree, almond butter, honey or maple syrup, pumpkin spice blend, and salt.
2. Mix until well combined.
3. Roll the mixture into balls and coat with chopped pecans if desired.
4. Refrigerate for at least 1 hour before serving.

65. Chocolate Avocado Mousse:

Preparation Time: 10 minutes
Nutrition:
   Calories: 150 per serving
   Protein: *3g*
   Carbohydrates: 12g
   Fat: 10g
Ingredients:
- 2 ripe avocados
- 1/4 cup cocoa powder
- 1/4 cup honey or maple syrup
- 1 teaspoon vanilla extract
- Pinch of salt
- Fresh berries for garnish

Instructions:
1. In a blender or food processor, combine ripe avocados, cocoa powder, honey or maple syrup, vanilla extract, and salt.
2. Blend until smooth and creamy.
3. Chill in the refrigerator for at least 2 hours before serving.
4. Garnish with fresh berries if desired.

66. Coconut and Almond Bliss Balls:

Preparation Time: 15 minutes
Nutrition:
  Calories: 100 per serving
  Protein: 2g
  Carbohydrates: 8g
  Fat: 7g
Ingredients:
- 1 cup shredded coconut
- 1/4 cup almond butter
- 2 tablespoons coconut oil, melted
- 2 tablespoons honey or maple syrup
- 1/2 teaspoon vanilla extract
- Pinch of salt
- **Instructions:**
- In a food processor, blend shredded coconut, almond butter, melted coconut oil, honey or maple syrup, vanilla extract, and salt until a dough forms.
- Roll the dough into small balls.
- Refrigerate for at least 1 hour before serving.

Feel free to customize these recipes based on your taste preferences, and enjoy these delightful grain-free sweet treats!

Conclusion

In concluding this Grain-Free Recipes Cookbook, our journey through a flavorful realm of wholesome, nutrient-dense, and delicious alternatives has been nothing short of extraordinary. We embarked on a culinary adventure, exploring the art of crafting meals that not only honor dietary choices but also celebrate the vibrant tapestry of ingredients available to us.

As we close the pages of this cookbook, we hope you've discovered that the absence of grains does not equate to a lack of taste or satisfaction. Instead, it opens the door to a world of creativity, where almond flour, coconut flour, and other grain-free ingredients serve as the palette for your culinary masterpiece.

Through seasonal specials that capture the essence of each time of year, ingredient spotlights that shed light on the benefits of key components, and personal insights from Dr. Olivia Fama's journey, we've strived to offer not just recipes but a holistic approach to a grain-free lifestyle.

In your hands, you hold more than a collection of recipes; you hold the power to transform your kitchen into a space of nourishment and joy. From breakfast to dessert, from soups to smoothies, we've aimed to provide a diverse array of options that cater to both the novice and the seasoned chef.

These recipes are not just about what you eat; they're about the experiences you create and share, the memories you forge, and the well-being you cultivate.

May this cookbook inspire you to experiment, to savor, and to relish the journey of grain-free living. As you embark on this culinary expedition, remember that each dish is a celebration of your commitment to health, and each bite is a testament to the incredible versatility and flavors that nature provides.

Thank you for allowing us to be a part of your kitchen, and here's to a future filled with delectable grain-free creations. May your cooking continue to be a source of joy, nourishment, and discovery. Cheers to a vibrant, flavorful, and grain-free life!

HAPPY COOKING

BONUS

MEALS PLANNER JOURNAL

Weekly Meal Planner Journal

Monday

Breakfast	
Lunch	
Dinner	

Tuesday

Breakfast	
Lunch	
Dinner	

Wednesday

Breakfast	
Lunch	
Dinner	

Thursday

Breakfast	
Lunch	
Dinner	

Friday

Breakfast	
Lunch	
Dinner	

Saturday

Breakfast	
Lunch	
Dinner	

Sunday

Breakfast	
Lunch	
Dinner	

Noted

Weekly Meal Planner Journal

Monday

Breakfast	
Lunch	
Dinner	

Tuesday

Breakfast	
Lunch	
Dinner	

Wednesday

Breakfast	
Lunch	
Dinner	

Thursday

Breakfast	
Lunch	
Dinner	

Friday

Breakfast	
Lunch	
Dinner	

Saturday

Breakfast	
Lunch	
Dinner	

Sunday

Breakfast	
Lunch	
Dinner	

Noted

Weekly Meal Planner Journal

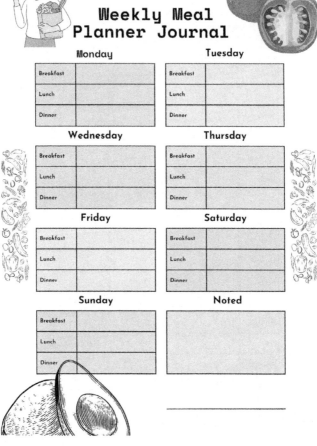

Monday

Breakfast	
Lunch	
Dinner	

Tuesday

Breakfast	
Lunch	
Dinner	

Wednesday

Breakfast	
Lunch	
Dinner	

Thursday

Breakfast	
Lunch	
Dinner	

Friday

Breakfast	
Lunch	
Dinner	

Saturday

Breakfast	
Lunch	
Dinner	

Sunday

Breakfast	
Lunch	
Dinner	

Noted

Weekly Meal Planner Journal

Monday

Breakfast	
Lunch	
Dinner	

Tuesday

Breakfast	
Lunch	
Dinner	

Wednesday

Breakfast	
Lunch	
Dinner	

Thursday

Breakfast	
Lunch	
Dinner	

Friday

Breakfast	
Lunch	
Dinner	

Saturday

Breakfast	
Lunch	
Dinner	

Sunday

Breakfast	
Lunch	
Dinner	

Noted

Weekly Meal Planner Journal

Monday

Breakfast	
Lunch	
Dinner	

Tuesday

Breakfast	
Lunch	
Dinner	

Wednesday

Breakfast	
Lunch	
Dinner	

Thursday

Breakfast	
Lunch	
Dinner	

Friday

Breakfast	
Lunch	
Dinner	

Saturday

Breakfast	
Lunch	
Dinner	

Sunday

Breakfast	
Lunch	
Dinner	

Noted

Weekly Meal Planner Journal

Monday

Breakfast	
Lunch	
Dinner	

Tuesday

Breakfast	
Lunch	
Dinner	

Wednesday

Breakfast	
Lunch	
Dinner	

Thursday

Breakfast	
Lunch	
Dinner	

Friday

Breakfast	
Lunch	
Dinner	

Saturday

Breakfast	
Lunch	
Dinner	

Sunday

Breakfast	
Lunch	
Dinner	

Noted

Weekly Meal Planner Journal

Monday

Breakfast	
Lunch	
Dinner	

Tuesday

Breakfast	
Lunch	
Dinner	

Wednesday

Breakfast	
Lunch	
Dinner	

Thursday

Breakfast	
Lunch	
Dinner	

Friday

Breakfast	
Lunch	
Dinner	

Saturday

Breakfast	
Lunch	
Dinner	

Sunday

Breakfast	
Lunch	
Dinner	

Noted

Printed in Great Britain
by Amazon